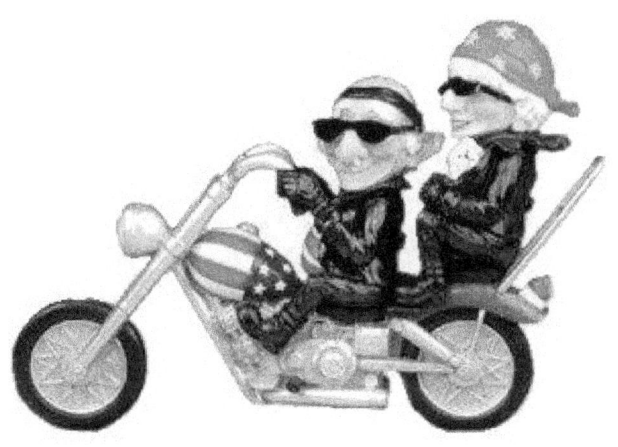

BABY BOOMERS
HEALTH & DIET

Gunter Schaule, BSc, MBA
Consulting Editor Dr U.de Brentani

© International Publishing

TABLE OF CONTENTS

Introduction

Exercise?

Excess Calories

Food Selection

Losing Weight – Explained

Detox

Spirit

Is it a Priority or Not?

Introduction

The Baby Boomers, born between the 1946 and 1964, have had a good run in life, and they want to keep it that way. You can't enjoy life without being healthy. Also, for the now ageing baby boomers, how long you live becomes a consideration at this stage.

A good deal of staying healthy depends on keeping your weight down. When we were younger, the body was more forgiving. But if we are overweight now, we are more likely to suffer the consequences, curses like diabetes, and crippling effects in the joints. Now, excess weight underlines our advancing age, whereas a trim body still bestows that young feeling on us. It has never been more important to control our weight than now.

This is where the secret of this eating plan comes in. Such a well kept secret: It is not difficult to control your weight. The trick is not how much you eat, but what you eat selectively across the whole food spectrum. This will be explained in detail later.

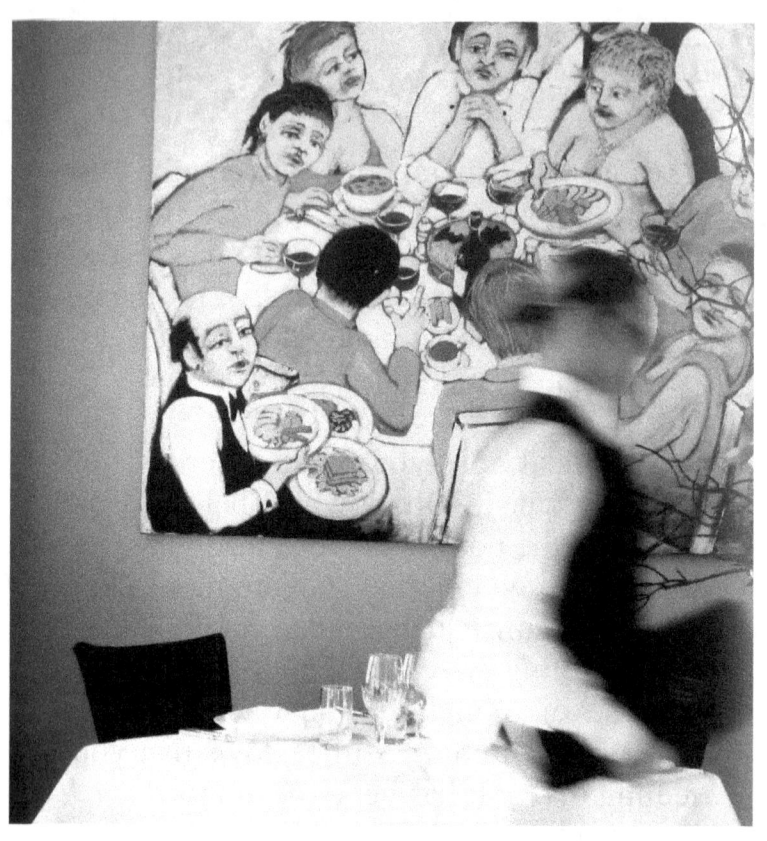

Exercise ?

Baby boomers were always strong on exercise, which is good, particularly for the cardiovascular system. One form, unfortunately, too much jogging, can be detrimental to the cartilages in the back bone and in the joints, which may catch up with some of us now. In any case, exercise requires serious and persistent efforts if it is meant to control body weight.

The fat burning effect of exercise can be overestimated.
For example, **½ an hour** of different types of exercises use up only the following calories on average:

Going for a walk burns just 75 cal.
Cycling in a flat area uses up 110 cal.
Light swimming in warm water 150 cal.
Moderate conditioning exercise 200 cal.
Jogging for half an hour burns 330 cal.

Yet, for example, eating some simple food adds the following:

One thick slice of white bread 100 cal.
A simple bowl of cornflakes 130 cal.
Just one bagel gives us 140 cal.
A serving of boiled pasta is 330 cal.
A serving of roasted potatoes 420 cal.

Modern exercise equipment displays the calories you are burning, which confirms the disappointing reality. So, if you want to keep or reduce your body weight, moderate exercise is only useful <u>without</u> additional eating or soft drinks. Only if you exercise intensely over longer periods of time, and if you have few body-fat reserves to burn, you require extra energy through additional food intake.

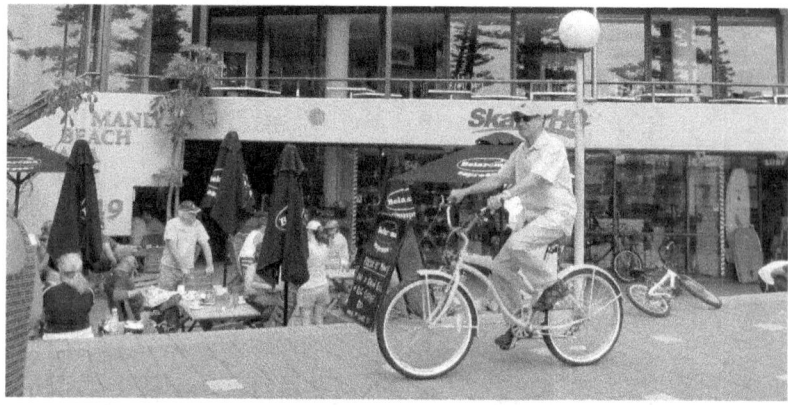

While many forms of exercise are good for our health, to lose weight it may be simpler to select food that gives you little extra energy, to make the body use the calories stored in body fat.

To keep it in perspective, compared to the exercise calories shown above, the body burns energy all the time, just to keep the system going, pumping blood, breathing, digesting food, and maintaining our body temperature. For an average person, that requires about 1400 calories a day. This is called the Basic Metabolic Rate (BMR). If you get out of bed, walk around the house and the office, sit at the PC, the TV, or in the car, that may add another 200 calories a day. That means:

Without any significant effort you burn about 1600 calories a day.

MUSCLE BUILDING RESISTANCE EXERCISE on a regular basis is particularly useful as we get older. It allows us to focus on our specific body weaknesses.

For example, if your stomach and back muscles need strengthening, lie on your back, bend your knees, and do sit-ups. Start with 20, and add a few more each time, until you reach over 100 per day. The simplest back exercise is to lie on your back, bring your legs back towards your buttocks and arch up your belly as high as you can. In this easy position, breathe deeply for a few minutes. Your back will get strong with little effort.

If your legs feel weak, do knee bends, or step-ups, or walk stairs every day.

As you get older, focus on your posture; this will help you to both feel and look younger.

Excess Calories

While we mentioned above not to take moderate exercise as an excuse for eating more, the main idea of the regime proposed here is not to eat less, but to eat the things which don't create more energy than we consume. Because our body stores excess energy as fat, as reserves for the days of famine. That trait harks back to the time of our ancestor cave dwellers. It helped them survive. Nowadays, in the developed world, famine is passé, we live in an overwhelming glut.

We are bombarded with food advertising, particularly for things that are not good for us, like cornflakes, orange juice and other things that are praised to give us energy. Which is fine if you are ploughing a field or cutting down trees. But most of us are sitting down more than anything else, at the PC, the TV, in the car. That requires little energy. Excess energy gets converted and stored as fat! This process will be explained later.

Kids eat an 'energy breakfast', and then they sit in school. After the fast energy spike, the excess gets stored away, and the kids get tired, their concentration wanes.

What most of us need is slow nutritional release, long lasting energy.

That's where food science springs to help. It tells us exactly what food items and drinks generate fast release or slow release energy.

And it tells us which food creates no energy at all. We can enjoy that type of nutrient just to build muscles, for example, or to satisfy our hunger feelings, or if we want to savour certain delicacies without penalties.

Science calls this magic food knowledge the 'Glycemic Index' (GI), a measure of the rise and subsequent decline in blood sugar levels produced by any food item.

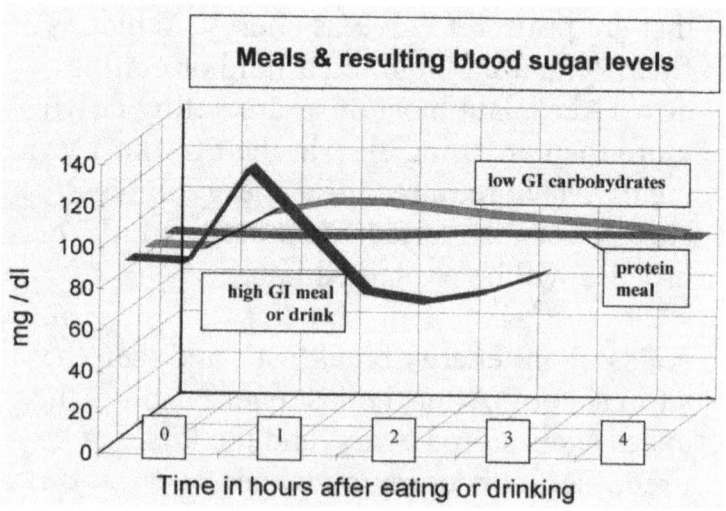

To consider the basic picture, we can look at the three main nutrients and their purpose:

Proteins (*e.g., meat, fish, cheese*)
build and maintain our body cells

Carbohydrates (*e.g., sugar, bread, potatoes*)
create energy & body reserves

Fats (*e.g., butter, oil, bacon*)
create reserves for future energy
production

Certain other important ingredients have
no calories
 e.g., water, fibers, minerals, vitamins

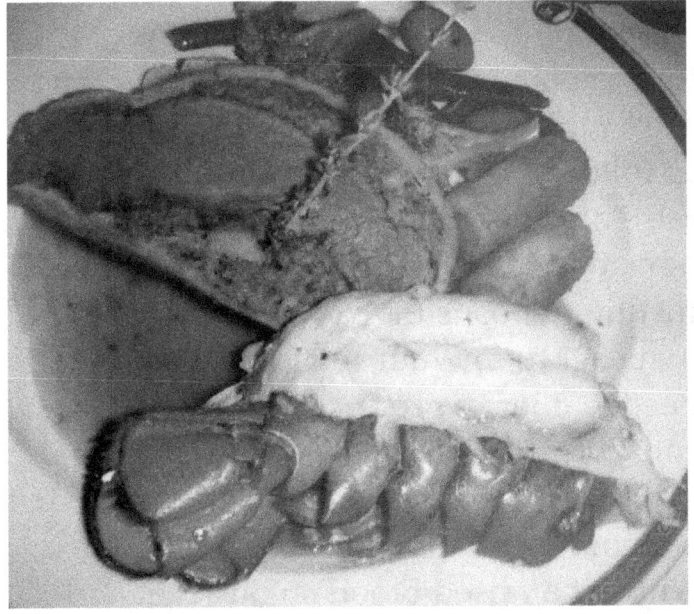

Excess calories in the form of *protein* get eliminated by the body. Our bodies simply cannot store proteins. But, energy producing *carbohydrates* are too vital to get wasted. Why? Our body is still built for the age-old experience of 'feast and famine'. Our body stores reserves for times of food scarcity. How? By converting certain carbohydrates into fat and by building fat pockets, it creates energy storage for future use. But nowadays, the famine part of the equation has dropped off the table. All that remains is the body fat, forever, and growing. Technically, the process works as follows. Some types of carbohydrates raise our blood sugar level, calling the hormone INSULIN into the blood stream. Insulin deposits the blood sugar (Glucagon) into our muscle cells for needed energy production, and it converts the excess into fat for storage purposes. Insulin also deposits the *fat* that is in our food into fat pockets. Therefore, without a raised blood sugar level and without increased Insulin, fat cannot be retained; it gets eliminated. Fat is only fattening if consumed with carbs that raise our blood sugar level.

The FIRST SECRET is: **Not all excess calories (e.g., proteins) get stored as fat.**

The SECOND SECRET is: **Only certain carbohydrates call enough Insulin into the blood stream to create fat pockets.**

It's important to realize that not all foods make us fat. As noted above, only certain types of carbohydrates are able to create fat pockets. So, the key question is: What kind of carbohydrates are these?

Only carbohydrates which raise our blood sugar to high levels quickly make us fat.

This effect is determined not only by their sugar content, but significantly by their cell structure that facilitates fast absorption in the digestive system.

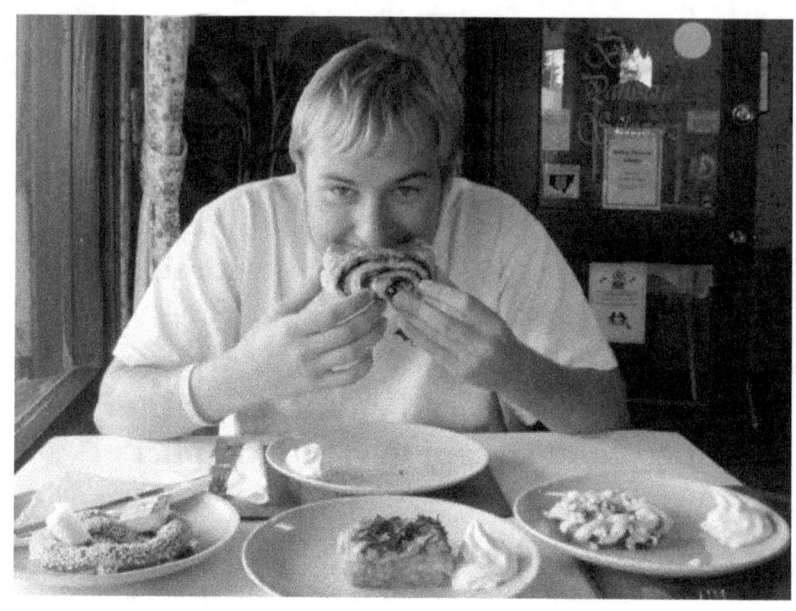

Food Selection

Below is a list of things you should never eat, because of their high GI value, or it should be considered as a sin for occasional transgressions only. It is a long list, but you won't miss that stuff, since there is another long list further down with all the goodies we should eat.

To control your weight, DON'T eat these:

Jasmine rice, GI 109
Dried dates, GI 103
Pancake mix, GI 102
French Baguette, GI 95
Instant rice, GI 91
Puffed rice, GI 90

Corn Thins, GI 87
Backed or mashed potatoes, GI 85
CORNFLAKES, GI 83
Rice cakes, GI 82
Jelly beans, GI 81
Wonderwhite TOAST, 80

Choco Pops, GI 77
Waffles, GI 76
Doughnut, GI 76
French fries, GI 75
Sports drink, GI 74
Sultana Bran Cereal, GI 73
Pop corn, GI 72
BAGLE, GI 72
Water cracker, GI 71
Wheatabix, GI 70

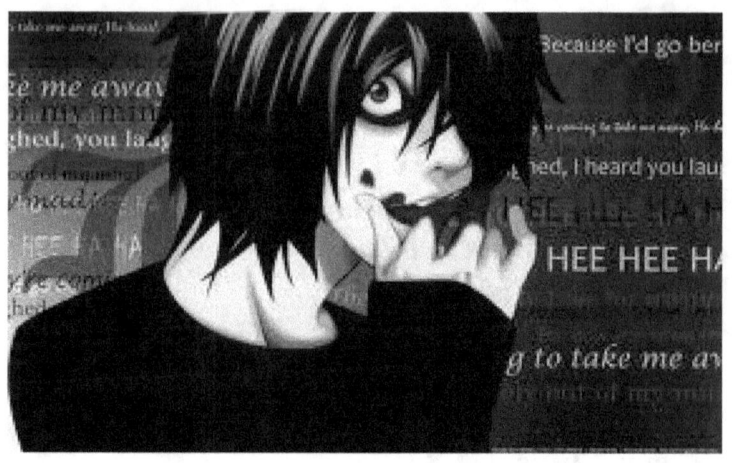

(Getting less detrimental with decreasing
GI, but recommended only occasionally:)

Cranberry juice, GI 68
Taco shell, GI 68
Special K cereal, GI 68
Croissant, GI 67
Nutri Grain, GI 66
Instant porridge, GI 66
Couscous, GI 65
Cantaloupe, GI 65
Beetroot, GI 64
White rice, GI 64
Raisins, GI 64
Shortbread, GI 64
Rey bread, GI 64
Coca Cola, GI 63

Ice cream, regular, GI 61
Hamburger bun, GI 61

Papaya, GI 59
Muffin or danish, GI 59
Orange juice, GI 57
Long grain rice, GI 56
Oat bran cereal, GI 55
Oatmeal cookies, GI 55
Sweet corn, GI 54
Sweet potato, GI 53
Banana, GI 52
Sushi roll, GI 52
Oranges, mango, kiwi fruit, GI 46
Pizza, macaroni, GI 46
Grapes, GI 46
Peaches, GI 42
Pumpernickel bread, GI 41

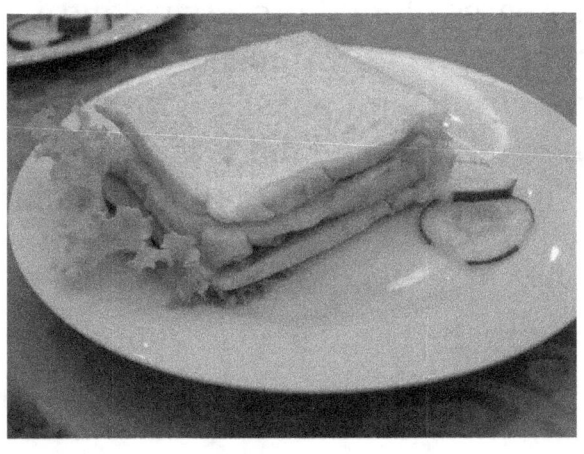

Seeing the everyday food in the table above, it may be hard to believe that this is the main problem! We are so used to these items, but we have to rethink our eating habits drastically to fit a lifestyle of everyday lower energy requirements.

If we want to lose weight, we must avoid everything listed above. It's not hard, it's just a question of knowing it. All we need for a healthy diet across all food categories we can find in the table below. From these items we can practically eat as much as we like. It is important to remind ourselves why there is such a wide range in GI values for carbohydrates. GI values depend on several things, including sugar content, degree of food processing and refinement (e.g. highly milled flower, processed cornflakes, polished rice with the bran removed), and importantly on the cell structure of the food (for example, potatoes get quickly digested by our body, and starch is converted to sugar and sent into the blood stream almost immediately, producing a lot of short-term energy).

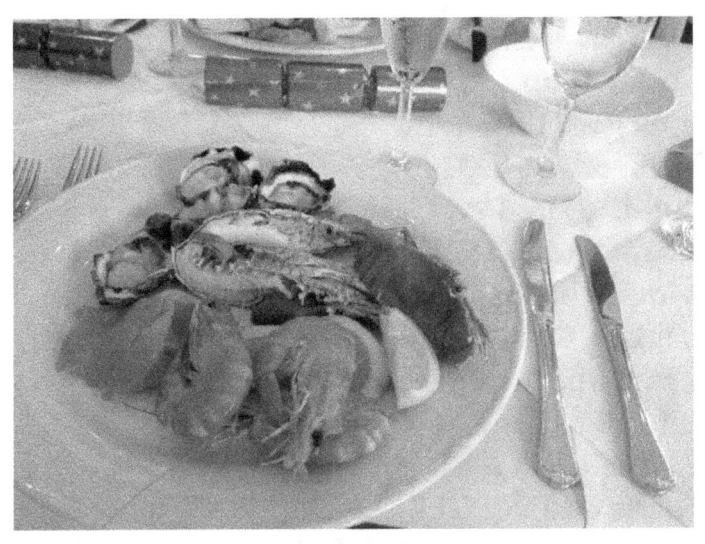

EAT AS MUCH AS YOU LIKE OF THIS

All Proteins –
**   – like meat, fish, cheese, GI 0 (zero)**
Water, dry wine, GI 0
Green beans, spinach, rocket, GI 0
Lettuce, celery, cucumber, GI 0
Avocado, GI 6
Mushrooms, GI 10
Broccoli, peppers, onions, GI 10
Natural plain yoghurt, GI 14
Peanuts, GI 14

Tomatoes, GI 15
Raw carrots, GI 16
Cashew nuts, GI 22
Cherries, GI 22
Milk, low fat, GI 24
Plums, GI 24
Grapefruit, GI 25
Kidney beans, GI 27
Lentils, GI 30
Dried apricots, GI 30
All Bran cereal, GI 30
Chickpeas, GI 36
Tomato juice, GI 38
Premium ice cream, GI 38
Apples, pears, GI 38
Strawberries, GI 39
Milk, soy milk, GI 40
Apple juice, GI 40

Even if the tables above are long, to provide a condensed view, the principle is quite simple:

Eat protein in a wide variety, together with salads and green vegetables, but without the starchy bulk fillers like potatoes, rice, bread and pasta.

For breakfast, forget the sugar laden orange juice, and artificially constituted cereals featuring in TV advertising.
"All Bran" is the only one with low sugar and high fibre. Better even, just oat bran from a generic package, mixed with yoghurt. Have smoked salmon, eggs, fried vegetables, even a steak if you are incredibly hungry. Forget toast, any bread and jam, danish, muffins and bagels.

Coffee is low GI, without sugar. It decreases the risk of Alzheimer's and it contains generally beneficial anti-oxidants.

Eat moderate climate fruit and berries, but not tropical fruits.

If you eat a hamburger, don't eat the bun, and certainly not the French fries!

In general, snack on low GI nibbles and fruits (see table above), to keep your blood sugar level and your energy level even throughout the day.

Forget all sweet drinks, like coke, lemonades, sports drinks, and sugary fruit juices. They give you a blood sugar spike that gets converted to fat, followed by an energy slump which leads to hunger pangs.

Dry wine is ok from a GI point of view, since all grape sugar has been converted into alcohol. It is a separate question to what extent the alcohol is healthy or not in other ways. All drugs need some self-control.

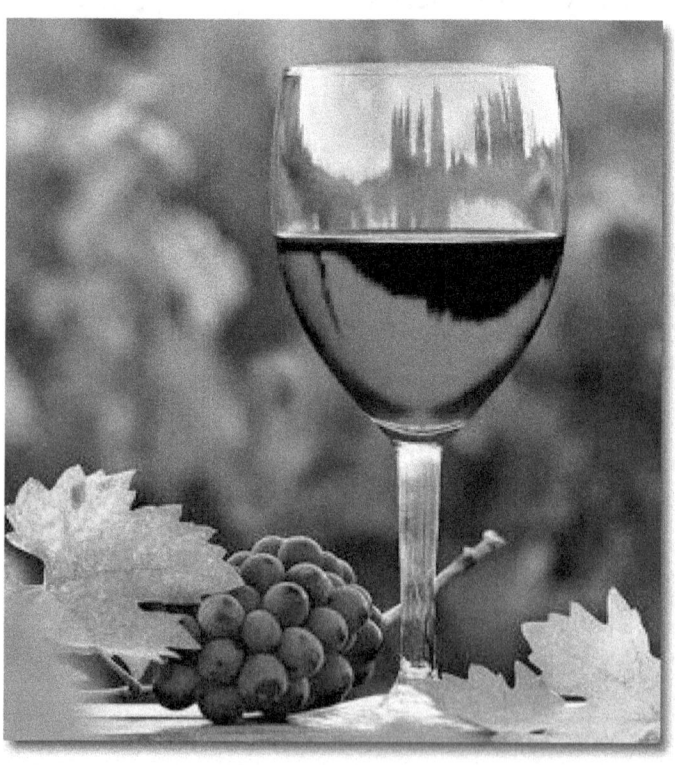

Losing Weight – Explained

So far we have been talking about a healthy diet to follow for a lifetime, to keep our weight down, or bring it down. Following here are further details describing the process. As noted, Insulin *deposits* blood sugar into cells. Once the blood sugar is down to its normal level and there is no more Insulin in the blood stream, the body looks elsewhere for energy. This is where another important hormone, called GLUCAGON, kicks in. Glucagon does exactly the opposite from Insulin; it *removes* fat from cells to produce energy. Therefore, shedding body fat doesn't start until a few hours after consuming carbohydrates - that is, when all the insulin has been absorbed. This means that you need to take extended breaks after high insulin producing meals if you want to lose weight. In other words, no sweet or starchy snacks, or sweet drinks, etc. between meals. But, because proteins produce no blood sugar and don't interfere with the fat burning action of Glucagon, you can enjoy other types of snacks such as cheese, eggs or meat cuts. Also, as shown in the GI table above, various kinds of salads have a GI of zero and are ideal snacks that don't prevent fat burning.

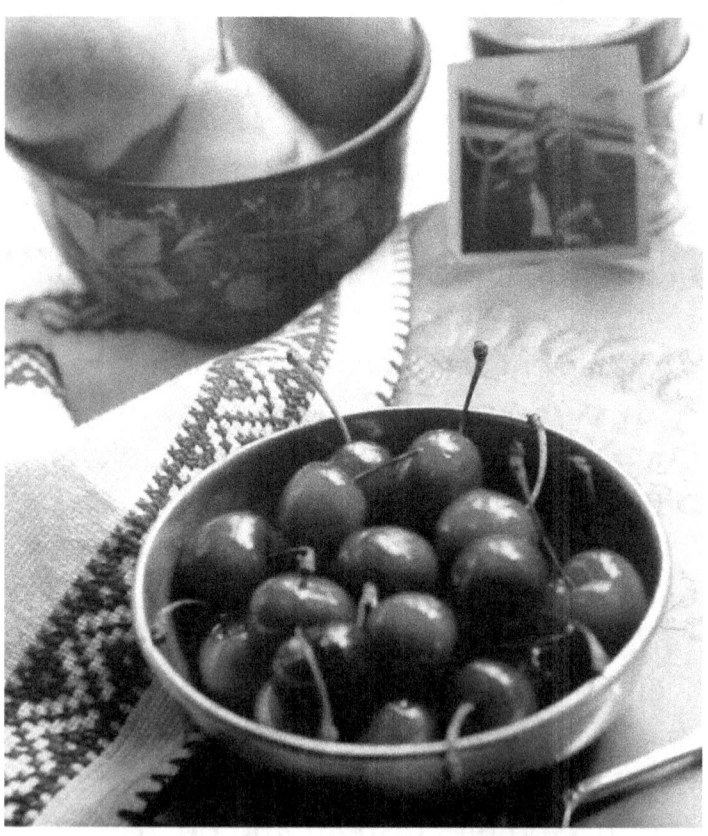

Let's look at how Insulin and Glucagon play each other off in our daily lives. At all times, day or night, our body needs energy for its basic functioning at the BMR. During the day, our level of energy use varies, depending on what we are doing. The more physically active we are, the faster the Insulin level decreases, and the sooner the Glucagon hormone gets released. So, the higher the level of activity, the earlier fat burning starts. Even at night, this fat burning action continues. While we are asleep, about 3 hours after our last carbohydrate meal, Glucagon starts burning fat. To get fat burning started earlier in the evening, it is important to avoid those last cookies, chocolates, or sweet nightcaps.

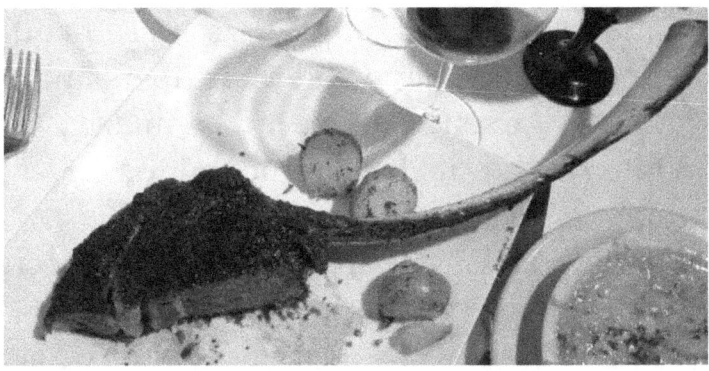

Detox

Another factor impacting our bodily health, and weight, is the level of acidity in our system. We speak of the need for 'detoxification'. A primary reason for toxification of our body is slow digestion and delayed bowel evacuation. The system slows down with age. This is a cause for concern.

Beside the toxifying effect, slow digestion also allows more food energy to be absorbed by the body, which leads to greater weight gain. The main reason for slow digestion is the highly processed nature of modern food. Finely milled flour, bread and breakfast cereals manufactured from highly processed and refined inputs, have had their fibers and natural coarseness removed. Similarly, white rice has its bran removed for appearance sake. As a result, the GI of many of our basic carbohydrates has been artificially increased to our detriment.

But even more devastating than causing slow digestion and therefore weight gain, the resulting waste product sits for too long in the last section of our intestines, the colon. There, it disseminates acidity and poisons our body. Cancer of the colon is the leading cause of death in men.

We need to eat more fibrous and less refined food — as our ancestors did — to stimulate our digestion. And if that is not enough, laxatives may be required. There are excellent natural laxatives on the market.

Detoxification through regular bowel movements - at least once a day - should be an important goal if you want to avoid cancer and stop poisoning your body with acidity.

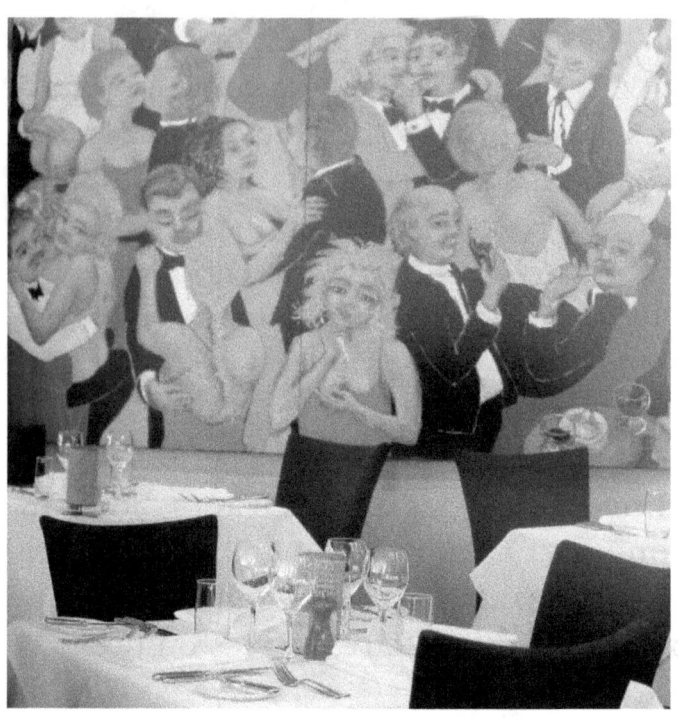

Various body processes may deteriorate as we get older. One of the most worrisome toxifications is that of the brain leading to ALZHEIMER'S.

Some surprising research has been published as of late regarding food and drink that slow down such memory decline:

COFFEE has been discovered as a tonic that decreases dementia-causing amyloid in the brain. And coffee contains beneficial anti-oxidants.

APPLE JUICE & APPLES motivate the generation of the memory chemical acetylcholine.

OMEGA 3 reduces plaque formations on blood vessels and keeps the blood flowing swiftly to all parts of the body, including the brain. Fish oil, flax seed oil and similar supplements provide extra Omega 3.

VITAMIN D deficiency is widespread amongst aging people, increasing the risk of cognitive impairment. Experts recommend vitamin D3 supplements.

AVOID INFECTIONS. All sorts of infections may migrate to the brain and wipe out brain cells, from gum infections to cold sores, gastric ulcers, Lyme decease, pneumonia and the flu. Use vaccines and antiviral agents.

BRAIN EXERCISE is vital. Use it or lose it. Learn new things. - Meditation also enhances cognitive functioning.

Spirit

The mood and the spirit of an experience have always been important to Baby Boomers. Happiness experts tell us that a key to feeling good is to appreciate what we encounter. They tell us to live in the present, to concentrate on our immediate environment and on our experiences as they happen. This advice applies well to eating and drinking. For each meal, we should select a conducive environment, admire the food presentation, and savor consciously every morsel and every drop we put into our mouth. Eating is a central activity of human social interaction, from family meals to intimate dates to great feasts and celebrations. Calorie counting and general abstinence inhibit and diminish such positive experiences. It is much wiser to eat selectively, based on the Glycemic Index (GI), thereby enjoying a wide variety and ample quantity of food and drink, without missing out on the fun and without gaining weight.

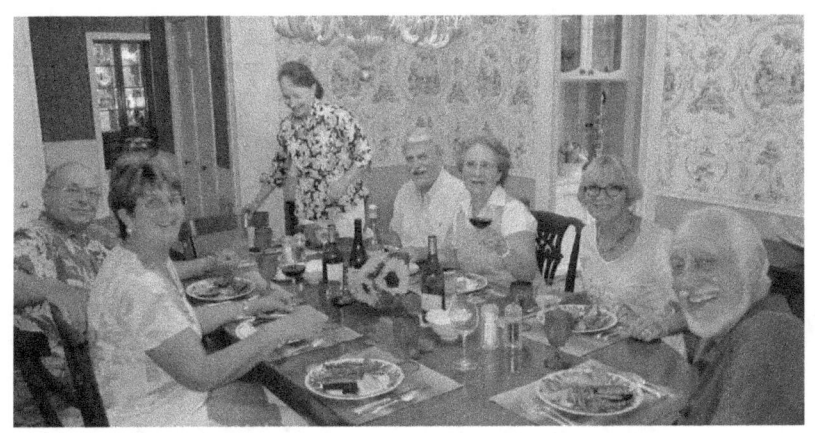

Is it a Priority or Not?

A frequent, quick and simple comment is,
'I can't live without eating my bread!'

You may put other words instead of bread
into this sentence, like potatoes, pasta, rice -
all the bulk fillers.

That is a question of priorities, whether you
accept overweight, joint problems, diabetes,
and cancer risk instead? It is a question of
how serious you actually are about your long-
term health.

The issue is simply, with what bodyweight and how long you want to live, and what you are willing to trade in for that reward.

Also, with advancing age, a trim body still bestows that young feeling on us. Balanced, sustained energy lifts the spirit.

The Baby Boomers, born between the 1946 and 1964, have had a good run in life, and they want to keep it that way for as long as possible!